Sex Energy Meditation

A simple guide to feeling more pleasure

Kathryn Peterson

www.kamakatyoga.com

Overview

My name is Kat and I am a private yoga teacher specializing in sex energy. I help my clients reduce stress, increase intimate connection, overcome sexual dysfunction, and enhance fertility. My work is called Kama Kat Yoga.

Kama means desire, pleasure, erotic love. Like in the Kama Sutra. The reason we desire something is because we believe that it will give us pleasure. The reason we desire something is because we don't yet have it. This desire, this longing, is key to erotic love. Because it's the tension of being apart that gives us the pleasure of coming together.

My clients who tend to struggle the most are those who don't realize the beauty of this tension. The beauty of desire. They see the longing as something negative, a hole that needs to be filled, that they are incomplete without that thing they desire.

When we realize that the longing is something positive, we feel pleasure in every moment. We realize that we are already filled and complete. Our journey is a pleasure. Our desire is a pleasure. And that thing is just expanding our pleasure, so we can take it all in deeper...

Sex energy meditation is how I learned to embody the pleasure of kama. I teach sex energy meditation to my clients so that they can learn to feel this pleasure too.

We use simple yoga exercises to move our sex energy from the root chakra to the heart chakra. This guide will give you a basic overview of these exercises and terms so that you can understand them immediately.

I encourage my clients to practice this meditation as part of their regular masturbation activity. Exploring different sensations of the erotic and of love. Feeling the bliss of a full-body orgasm. Allowing ourselves to be overcome with the joy of kama.

You will be able to practice sex energy meditation immediately after reading this guide. Remember that even if you start training for a marathon today, you probably won't be ready for the race tomorrow. But every day you get closer. And when our training is in sex energy meditation, every day you will feel even more pleasure.

Sex Energy

When he touches my arm and my whole body feels warm and tingling. Like I'm melting into the ground beneath his hands. Longing to feel him rub me up and down...

Sex energy is that feeling of electric ecstasy.
It's not about what you do.
It's about what you feel.

Because anyone could touch your arm,
but it feels different when your lover touches your arm.

An easy way to feel your sex energy is when you are aroused. That sensation of arousal is your sex energy activating. Sex energy meditation is easiest to practice during masturbation because you can focus on that feeling without distraction.

Try masturbating with the intention of becoming aware of your sex energy…

What are the sensations of sex energy in your body?
Maybe you are feeling more relaxed.
Maybe you are feeling more excited.
Maybe you are feeling hotter.

How do these sensations change as you climax?
Maybe you are feeling a stronger burning.
Maybe you are feeling a deeper pulsing.
Maybe you are feeling a rush.

Where does your sex energy go after climax?
Maybe you are feeling it release between your legs.
Maybe you are feeling it drip down into your toes.
Maybe you are feeling it expand inside of you…

Yoga

Yoga is about opening up so that there is more space for breath to circulate. And breath is life.

Prana is what we call breath in yoga.
Prana is life force energy.

Yoga activates the parasympathetic nervous system, which puts the brakes on the stress response. Research suggests that mindful breathing is how yoga reduces stress.

Pranayama is how we mindfully breathe in yoga.

Mindfulness is about awareness,
simply noticing what we think and feel,
without becoming what we think and feel.

When we are chronically stressed, our body is chronically producing stress hormones like cortisol. This inhibits our body from producing sex hormones like testosterone and estrogen. Higher testosterone increases male libido. Higher estrogen increases female libido. Higher cortisol decreases all libido.

By reducing stress,
we restore our hormonal balance.

By increasing mindfulness,
we feel our pleasure more deeply.

Pranayama

Pranayama means intentionally flowing the vital life force.

Breathe in through your nose.
Breathe out through your mouth.

Now place your hands around your belly button.
When you inhale through your nose, expand your belly.
When you exhale through your mouth, release your belly.

Let's try a simple pranayama exercise called belly breathing.
Our intention is to regulate our breath for a count of six
but you can work your way up. Let's practice.

We inhale through our nose, expanding the belly.
We exhale through our mouth, releasing the belly.

Inhale, 2, 3.
Exhale, 2, 3.

Inhale, 2, 3, 4
Exhale, 2, 3, 4.

Inhale, 2, 3, 4, 5.
Exhale, 2, 3, 4, 5.

Inhale, 2, 3, 4, 5, 6.
Exhale, 2, 3, 4, 5, 6.

Try practicing pranayama for five minutes...

Inhaling and expanding your belly, 2, 3, 4, 5, 6.
Exhaling and releasing your belly, 2, 3, 4, 5, 6.

Vibrational Frequency

Let's say that you're longing to have sex, but your partner seems to be losing interest. Maybe your partner isn't interested in sex with you at all. You try asking, coercing, begging. And every night your resentment builds along with your desire...

Let's say that you're longing to have an orgasm. You try different positions, different toys, different angles. You get worked up to excitement, but never have you felt that elusive wave of bliss coming over and through your being...

Let's say that you're longing to have an intimate connection. You meet plenty of partners that pleasure you physically, socially, intellectually. But still it feels like something is missing. That desire to be pleasured soulfully lies forever untouched by another...

Lack of sex.
Lack of orgasm.
Lack of intimacy.

Our problem is the vibrational frequency of lack.

When I say vibration, I mean the vibration of the cells in our body. They create an electromagnetic field that travels by waves. Our vibrational frequency refers to how fast these waves move.

Low frequency vibrations (under 100Hz) are associated with feelings of fear, apathy, longing. Feelings that make us contract. Vibrations of lack that attract more lack.

High frequency vibrations (over 500Hz) are associated with energies of love, peace, joy. Feelings that make us expand. Vibrations of abundance that attract more abundance.

Like how a radio brings you different music. Just because the radio is not playing jazz music right now, does not mean that a jazz station does not exist. It simply means that you are not tuned to its frequency. You receive jazz music once you are in tune to the jazz channel.

If I want to feel dripping with the passion of my deep erotic ocean. That my body, mind, and soul are exploding with waves of ecstasy. I cannot be in tune to the feelings of resentment, disappointment, or resentment. I must be in tune to that channel of overflowing pleasure and fulfillment...

Our solution is the vibrational frequency of abundance.

Sex Energy Meditation

Mindfulness and meditation are both about awareness. Mindfulness is a general approach, while meditation is a specific practice. Like how vegetarianism is a general approach to eating, while oats and berries for breakfast is a specific practice of that eating.

Sex energy meditation is a specific practice for moving our sex energy from the root chakra at our genitals to the heart chakra at our chest.

Chakras are what we call energy centers in yoga.
The main chakra system moves along the spine.

The lower chakras at the bottom of the spine are associated with lower vibrational frequencies. They are not vibrational frequencies that make us shrink but simply are vibrational frequencies that connect us to the physical world. Security, creativity, identity.

The higher chakras at the top of the spine are associated with higher vibrational frequencies. These vibrational frequencies expand us beyond the physical world and connect us to the spiritual world. Truth, wisdom, enlightenment. The world of pure joy.

The Root Chakra

The root chakra is located at the pelvic floor. The pelvic floor is made up of the muscles and tissue that line the pelvis. It holds our bladder, rectum, and reproductive organs.

The root chakra is associated with our physical life. For all of us were created by the sex organs of our parents.

The center of the pelvic floor is located at the perineum, the area between the genitals and the anus. Some people call it the taint. Yogis call it the third foot, because we want to point it between our other two feet. Planting our root.

A simple way to activate your pelvic floor is imagine that you are urinating and that you have to stop the flow mid-stream. It's like you are pulling your perineum up towards your head. Those muscles contracting are the pelvic floor.

Mulabandha is how we mindfully activate the pelvic floor in yoga.

Mindfully activating the pelvic floor is how we can physically pump fluids to and from our genitals. Our genitals are made of erectile tissue, engorging with blood and giving us the sensation of arousal. Pumping blood to the genitals is how we can expand our arousal.

Pelvic floor activation is key to semen retention for men. Ejaculation is a physiological response while orgasm is an energetic response. Building the pelvic floor muscles strong enough to hold back ejaculation, is how men can experience the bliss of multiple orgasms.

Mindfully activating the pelvic floor is how we can metaphysically pump sex energy to and from our genitals.

When we mindlessly dump our sex energy outside of ourself, sex depletes us. It's why you get tired after having sex. Because all that power, the energy that creates life, the energy that creates love, flew out from between your legs, right into the ether.

When we mindfully circulate our sex energy inside of ourself, sex elevates us. Moving sex energy up the spine, up the chakra system, is how we can expand that electric sensation and elation inside of our self. It's how we feel the pleasure of a full-body orgasm. It's how we raise our vibrational frequency. It's how we transform lust into love.

Mulabandha

Mulabandha means locking the root chakra.

Firstly, make sure that your pelvic floor is in the anatomically correct alignment. Remember that the perineum is the center of the pelvic floor. Make sure that your perineum is pointing between your legs. If you are sitting, sit on top of your perineum.

Secondly, start activating your pelvic floor. Remember that the feeling of contracting your pelvic floor is like you are pulling your perineum towards your head. Try contracting your pelvic floor right now.

Thirdly, synchronize your breath with your pelvic floor contraction. Inhale as you contract your pelvic floor. Exhale as you release your pelvic floor. Try practicing this right now.

Inhale & contract.
Exhale & release.

Inhale & contract.
Exhale & release.

Inhale & contract.
Exhale & release.

Then we can go deeper by expanding our breath along with our pelvic floor movement. Slowly inhaling while gradually contracting your pelvic floor. Slowly exhaling while gradually releasing your pelvic floor. Try it for a count of three.

Inhale & contract, 2, 3.
Exhale & release, 2, 3.

Inhale & contract, 2, 3.
Exhale & release, 2, 3.

Inhale & contract, 2, 3.
Exhale & release, 2, 3.

Try practicing mulabandha for five minutes...

Inhaling and contracting your pelvic floor, 2, 3.
Exhaling and releasing your pelvic floor, 2, 3.

The Heart Chakra

The heart chakra is located at the chest: the middle of the 7 chakras, the bridge between the physical and spiritual worlds.

The heart chakra is associated with love. But the problem is that many of us confuse love with ego validation.

Love is about allowing things to unfold naturally, trusting the divine timing of the universe.

Ego validation is about controlling things to go the way that we think they should go, because we think we know better than the universe.

Love is a flowing.
Love is a feeling.

Ego is a forcing and you can't force a feeling...

Sex Energy Meditation: Guided Practice

I love to practice at night
when everyone else is sleeping,
when it's just me and the moon.

I bathe and then lay in bed
rubbing coconut oil all over
my legs, arms, back, and chest.

My skin soft.
My spirit soft.
My breath soft.

I start with my pranayama...
Inhale and expand, 2, 3, 4, 5, 6.
Exhale and release, 2, 3, 4, 5, 6.

Rubbing slowly with each breath.
Sometimes remembering what his hands feel like.
Sometimes trying to forget him and just feel me.

Feeling the suppleness, the throbbing,
the rush of pleasure washing over me.

I breathe even deeper...
Inhale and expand, 2, 3, 4, 5, 6, 7, 8, 9.
Exhale and release, 2, 3, 4, 5, 6, 7, 8, 9.

Feeling the flame of desire blazing between my legs.
Burning and yearning to explode right now.

When we feel that urgency to go fast is
when we need to slow down and let it expand.

I start with my mulabandha…
Inhale and contract, 2, 3.
Exhale and release, 2, 3.

The heat spreads through me with every contraction.
From the root chakra at my genitals, to the sacral chakra at
back of my waist, to the solar plexus chakra above my belly
button, filling me all the way up to the heart chakra at my
chest.

There aren't any problems to be solved.
There are only problems to be dis-solved.

My problem was that he isn't here right now.
But I feel my whole body pulsing already.
But I feel my heart growing inside me already.

I become one with my mulabandha…Inhale and contract,
feeling my sex energy shoot up to my heart. Exhale and
release, feeling my sex energy drip down to my genitals.

Every breath an explosion of that desire inside me.

I melt into my pleasure under the light of the moon.

Sex Energy Meditation: Your Simple Practice

Try practicing sex energy meditation for 30 minutes...

Your intention is to flow your sex energy from the root chakra to the heart chakra.

Practice masturbation to help you feel your sex energy.

Practice pranayama to help you relax.

Practice mulabandha to help you feel your flow.

Practice becoming your pleasure...

Thank You

Thank you for reading this sex energy meditation guide.

Sex energy meditation is how I learned to let go.
Sex energy meditation is how I teach my clients to let go.
Sex energy meditation is how you can learn to let go...

Remember that the more you try to reach an orgasm, a certain outcome in a certain way, is when it starts to feel impossible. But when you finally relax and feel the rapture, letting go of all the stress and the forcing, letting yourself be free. That's when the peak of pleasure comes to you.

It's not about letting go of the desire so that we can accept a life of emptiness. It's not about lack.

It's about letting go of the desire so that we can accept a life of fullness beyond the desire. It's about abundance.

If you have any questions about sex energy meditation. If you would like to learn more about my work...

www.kamakatyoga.com

Made in the USA
Middletown, DE
23 September 2025